ECZEMA DIET COOKBOOK

Delicious Anti-Inflammatory Recipes To Heal Your Skin, Reduce Flare-Ups, And Improve Gut Health

DR ELIAN GRIFFIN

DISCLAIMER

The nutritional recommendations and recipes in this book are meant solely for informative reasons. They are not meant to replace the counsel, diagnosis, or care of a qualified medical expert. If you have any doubts about a medical condition or dietary requirements, you should always see your physician or another trained healthcare expert.

All reasonable efforts have been taken by the author and publisher to ensure that the information contained in this book is correct as of the date of publication. Recommendations may alter, though, as medical knowledge is always changing. When using any of the recipes or instructions found here, the user assumes all liability and assumes no risk, whether personal or otherwise. People who have certain dietary requirements or medical issues should speak with a healthcare provider for personalized guidance. The given recipes are only ideas; you may need to adjust them to suit your own nutritional needs, tastes, and tolerances.

When you use this book, you agree to release the publisher, the author, and their representatives from any liability for any claims, damages, liabilities, costs, or expenditures resulting from your use of the book.

TABLE OF CONTENTS

ABOUT THE BOOK

"Eczema Diet Cookbook" is an essential resource for anyone looking to control and reduce eczema symptoms by making dietary changes. The book starts with an introduction that goes into detail about eczema, its causes, and the important role diet plays in influencing its symptoms. It also shows how certain foods can either exacerbate or lessen eczema and provides information on how this cookbook can help readers make effective dietary changes. Finally, it includes advice on how to successfully follow the eczema diet, as well as answers to frequently asked questions and common concerns. All of these details set the stage for a thorough journey toward better skin health.

This book provides a thorough understanding of the fundamentals of eczema and its different forms, highlighting the role that diet plays in controlling symptoms. It also highlights the significance of identifying trigger foods and elucidates the direct relationship between diet and skin health. The book also includes advice on how to begin an eczema diet plan, so that readers can make well-informed dietary decisions.

A smooth transition to an eczema-friendly diet is ensured by providing sample meal plans, beginner-friendly recipes, and strategies for meal prepping, especially for those with busy schedules. Creating meal plans, understanding food labels, and navigating grocery shopping are all made simple with these comprehensive steps.

A complete list of eczema-friendly ingredients is provided, along with essential foods that support an eczema diet and those to avoid. Anti-inflammatory foods, drinking plenty of water, and thinking about nutritional supplements for skin health are all covered in detail.

In addition, the book includes healthy cooking methods that retain nutrients, flavor enhancement with herbs and spices that don't irritate the skin, and quick and simple recipes that fit into an eczema-friendly diet.

Practical and inclusive meal preparation is ensured by the book's tips for batch cooking, freezing, and feeding family members with varying dietary requirements.

The book provides eczema sufferers with healthy breakfast and snack options, such as nutrient-rich smoothies and dairy-free, gluten-free snack ideas. It also addresses how to control cravings without making eczema worse, giving readers a wide range of options that will satisfy their skin.

Flavorful salads, soups, stews, one-pot meals, plant-based dishes, and protein-rich options are among the lunch and dinner recipes that are designed to calm the skin and are simple to make. Desserts and treats that prevent flare-ups of eczema are also included so that readers can enjoy a variety of meals without sacrificing the health of their skin.

Holidays and special occasions can be difficult for eczema sufferers to manage, but this cookbook provides ideas for eczema-friendly entertaining and holiday meal modifications.

Dessert recipes, advice on dining out, and stress-reduction techniques are all included to help readers enjoy these occasions without worrying about flare-ups.

The book highlights the significance of complementary skincare routines, stress management, the impact of exercise and sleep on skin health, and the role that lifestyle modifications play in managing eczema. Holistic approaches to managing eczema are also explored, offering a comprehensive approach to treatment.

The book addresses common issues with adhering to an eczema diet and offers troubleshooting tips for those who are still having flare-ups despite following dietary changes. It also offers advice on how to modify recipes to suit individual tastes, get professional advice, and deal with concerns regarding dietary restrictions.

The book guides how to monitor symptoms and dietary effects, reintroduce foods after symptom improvement, and create a sustainable eczema-friendly lifestyle.

CHAPTER ONE

KNOWING THE CAUSES OF ECZEMA AND HOW FOOD AFFECTS SYMPTOMS

The chronic skin condition known as eczema, also called atopic dermatitis, is characterized by red, irritated, and itchy patches of skin. It is believed to be caused by a combination of genetic and environmental factors, and triggers can include allergens, irritants, stress, and hormonal changes. Patients with eczema have compromised skin barriers, which increases sensitivity and susceptibility to inflammation. Eczema often starts in childhood, but it can affect people of any age.

Food is a major factor in controlling eczema symptoms because certain foods can either cause flare-ups or help prevent them. Dairy products, eggs, nuts, wheat, and soy are examples of common triggers. On the other hand, including anti-inflammatory foods high in omega-

3 fatty acids, like fish, flaxseeds, and leafy greens, can help reduce inflammation and support skin health. Knowledge of these dietary effects enables people to make decisions that can positively influence their eczema symptoms.

To address eczema with food, it's critical to maintain a food journal to pinpoint individual triggers and patterns. Health professionals may prescribe elimination diets to identify particular food allergens or sensitivities. By being aware of the connection between food and eczema, people can take proactive measures to manage their condition and enhance their quality of life.

DIET IS IMPORTANT FOR MANAGING ECZEMA

It is impossible to overestimate the role that diet plays in managing eczema. For many people with eczema, eating certain foods can either cause or worsen symptoms, which increase inflammation, itching, and discomfort. By following an eczema-friendly diet, people can greatly lower the frequency and intensity of flare-ups, which in turn improves their overall skin health and quality of life.

A diet designed to manage eczema usually emphasizes nutrient-dense, anti-inflammatory options while avoiding common trigger foods. This means including lots of fruits and vegetables, lean proteins, and foods high in essential fatty acids. Omega-3 fatty acids, which are found in flaxseeds, walnuts, and salmon as well as other fish, have been shown to help reduce inflammation in the body, including the skin.

Vitamins and minerals like vitamin E, vitamin C, zinc, and selenium are vital for skin health and repair and should be prioritized in an eczema-friendly diet. By avoiding known triggers and prioritizing these nutrients, people can effectively manage their eczema and minimize its impact on their daily lives. Additionally, keeping a balanced diet supports immune system integrity and supports the integrity of the skin barrier.

With a focus on supporting skin health and reducing inflammation, the "Eczema Diet Cookbook" offers a variety of tasty and nutritious recipes that are specifically tailored to manage eczema through diet. Each recipe is carefully crafted to exclude common trigger foods while incorporating ingredients known for their anti-inflammatory properties.

With this cookbook, people can experiment with a variety of satisfying and skin-healthy meal options. From antioxidant-rich breakfasts to hearty dinners full of omega-3s, there's something for every taste and dietary requirement. The recipes are simple to follow, with step-by-step instructions and ingredient lists that make meal planning fun and easy.

In addition to recipes, the cookbook offers helpful advice on grocery shopping, meal planning, and keeping up a healthy eating schedule. It equips people with the information and resources they need to make educated decisions about their diet and how it affects their eczema symptoms. By adopting the principles and recipes in this cookbook, people can take charge of their eczema and improve the health of their skin.

ADVICE FOR USING THE ECZEMA DIET COOKBOOK SUCCESSFULLY

It takes commitment and planning to effectively manage eczema with food. The following useful advice will help you get the most out of the "Eczema Diet Cookbook" and make the most of it:

Firstly, familiarize yourself with the cookbook's guidelines and recommended foods. Understanding which ingredients to include and which to avoid will help you plan meals effectively. Keep a food diary to track your intake and monitor any potential triggers or improvements in your symptoms. This will enable you to identify patterns and make adjustments as needed. Experiment with different recipes and meal combinations to find what works best for your taste preferences and dietary needs. Variety ensures you stay motivated and satisfied with your meals. Stay consistent with your dietary changes. Consistency is key to seeing long-term improvements in eczema symptoms. Stick to the recommended guidelines and give your body time to respond positively to the changes. Consult with a healthcare professional or a nutritionist if you have specific dietary concerns or medical conditions that may impact your diet choices. They can provide personalized advice and support to help you achieve your health goals. By following these tips, you can effectively integrate the "Eczema Diet Cookbook" into your daily routine and experience the positive effects of a skin-supportive diet.

COMMON QUESTIONS AND ANSWERS REGARDING DIET AND ECZEMA

Here are some frequently asked questions (FAQs) to assist dispel uncertainties and offer helpful information when navigating eczema and its nutritional consequences.

Can a diet be used to treat eczema alone? Although diet helps control the condition's symptoms, it is not a cure for eczema, which is a complex disorder influenced by immune responses, environment, and heredity. Eating a diet that is eczema-friendly can help minimize flare-ups and improve skin health.

It varies from person to person, so maintaining a food diary and getting tested for allergies can help uncover personal triggers. Common trigger foods for eczema include dairy products, eggs, nuts, wheat, soy, and some fruits and vegetables.

Yes, diets high in antioxidants (found in fruits and vegetables), omega-3 fatty acids (found in fish and flaxseeds), and foods that support gut health (found in probiotics) can help reduce inflammation and support skin integrity. These foods can also help alleviate the symptoms of eczema.

Individual responses vary, but many people experience improvements in their eczema symptoms within a few weeks to a few months after implementing an eczema-friendly diet. Long-term benefits are contingent upon consistency and adherence to dietary recommendations.

Should I speak with a doctor before changing my diet to treat my eczema? Speaking with a doctor is advised before making any major dietary changes. A dermatologist or nutritionist, in particular, can offer tailored advice based on your unique condition, medical history, and dietary preferences.

People can feel more confident and knowledgeable about controlling their eczema through food choices by answering these often-asked questions and offering straightforward, helpful solutions. This information enables people to take proactive measures toward better skin and general well-being.

CHAPTER TWO

FUNDAMENTALS OF DIET AND ECZEMA

WHAT ARE THE COMMON TYPES OF ECZEMA?

Eczema, also called atopic dermatitis, is a chronic skin condition that mostly affects people in their early childhood but can affect people at any age. There are several types of eczema, each with its unique characteristics. Atopic dermatitis is the most common type and is frequently associated with allergies and asthma. Contact dermatitis is caused by skin contact with irritants or allergens. Dyshidrotic eczema causes itchy blisters on the palms, fingers, and soles of the feet. Nummular eczema appears as circular patches of irritated skin, while seborrheic dermatitis mainly affects areas rich in oil glands, like the face and scalp.

While symptoms can vary, common features include redness, dryness, itching, and inflammation. Treatment typically entails moisturizing the skin, avoiding triggers, and using prescribed medications like corticosteroids to reduce inflammation. Understanding these types is crucial for proper diagnosis and management.

DIETARY FACTORS IN CONTROLLING ECZEMA SYMPTOMS

The management of eczema symptoms is greatly influenced by diet, as certain foods can either precipitate flare-ups or worsen pre-existing symptoms. Although individual trigger foods differ, common culprits include dairy products, eggs, nuts, wheat, and soy. These foods can cause allergic reactions or sensitivities that present as itchy, inflammatory skin. Creating an eczema-friendly diet entails identifying and removing these trigger foods while emphasizing nutrient-dense, anti-inflammatory foods.

To support overall skin health and potentially reduce inflammation associated with eczema, an eczema diet typically consists of whole, unprocessed foods rich in antioxidants, vitamins, and minerals; staples include fresh fruits and vegetables, lean proteins like fish and poultry, and healthy fats from sources like avocados and olive oil. Steering clear of processed foods, sugary snacks, and excessive caffeine can also be beneficial for those managing eczema symptoms.

Effectively managing eczema requires knowing which foods to avoid. Since trigger foods can differ greatly from person to person, it's important to record flare-ups after particular meals in a food diary. Common triggers include dairy products, gluten-containing foods, shellfish, and some fruits, like citrus. These foods can cause allergic reactions or sensitivities that worsen eczema symptoms, like itching, redness, and inflammation.

A balanced diet can be achieved while identifying specific triggers; once trigger foods are identified, people can modify their diet to support skin health and minimize eczema symptoms. Reducing the frequency and severity of eczema flare-ups can be achieved by eliminating trigger foods from your diet. This process often involves an elimination diet, where suspected trigger foods are removed for some time, and then gradually reintroduced to observe reactions. Working with a healthcare professional or registered dietitian can streamline this process, ensuring a balanced diet while identifying specific triggers.

DIETARY FACTORS AND SKIN HEALTH

Skin health is greatly influenced by diet; it affects the look, feel, and general health of the skin. Diets high in processed foods, sugars, and unhealthy fats can exacerbate skin conditions like eczema, acne, and dryness. On the other hand, diets high in antioxidants, omega-3 fatty acids, and essential nutrients support healthy skin by promoting cell regeneration and reducing inflammation.

Antioxidant-rich foods like berries, tomatoes, and dark chocolate fight oxidative stress, which can speed up skin aging and exacerbate conditions like eczema. Vitamin C, found in citrus fruits and leafy greens, supports collagen production and skin repair. Vitamin E, found in nuts and seeds, acts as an antioxidant, protecting skin cells from damage. Omega-3 fatty acids, found in fatty fish like salmon and walnuts, help maintain skin moisture and reduce inflammation.

A well-balanced diet that emphasizes whole foods and minimizes processed snacks and sugary drinks can improve skin health and lessen the symptoms of eczema.

Staying hydrated is also important; drinking enough water helps the skin stay hydrated and function as a whole. People can take control of their skin health and prevent diseases like eczema by knowing how their food choices affect their skin.

BEGINNING THE ECZEMA DIET REGIMEN

Beginning an eczema diet plan entails thoughtful meal planning and mindful food selections to support skin health and effectively manage symptoms. Start by focusing on nutrient-dense, anti-inflammatory foods like fresh fruits and vegetables, lean proteins, and healthy fats like avocado and olive oil, and identifying trigger foods through a food diary or elimination diet, eliminating potential allergens or sensitivities.

A registered dietitian or healthcare provider can help you create a customized diet plan that meets your nutritional needs and addresses your eczema symptoms. Meal preparation is crucial; incorporate eczema-friendly recipes that prioritize whole ingredients and steer clear of processed foods, artificial additives, and excessive sugars. Try out allergen-free alternatives for common triggers like dairy and gluten to maintain variety and flavor in your diet while minimizing flare-ups.

Maintaining a consistent diet plan is essential for improving the overall health of your skin and managing symptoms of eczema. You should also keep an eye on how your skin responds to dietary modifications and modify your meal plan as necessary to get the best results. People with eczema can support their skin's natural healing process and enjoy healthier, more comfortable skin by eating a balanced, eczema-conscious diet and making educated food choices.

CHAPTER THREE

HOW TO MAKE A MEAL PLAN THAT IS ECZEMA-FRIENDLY

Planning meals that include plenty of antioxidants and vital nutrients like vitamins A, C, and E, which promote skin health and repair, is the first step in creating an eczema-friendly meal plan.

Focus on whole, unprocessed foods rich in anti-inflammatory properties like fruits, vegetables, lean proteins, and healthy fats. These foods help reduce inflammation, a common trigger for eczema flare-ups.

To help you identify triggers more effectively, keep a food diary to track how different foods affect your skin. Make sure your meals are balanced, incorporating a variety of colors and textures to provide a spectrum of nutrients. Experiment with cooking methods that retain nutrients while avoiding excessive oils or frying, which can introduce skin-irritating compounds. Rotate your ingredients when planning meals to avoid potential allergens and sensitivities.

Last but not least, customize your meal plan to fit your tastes and lifestyle. Make meals ahead of time to save stress and temptations at the last minute. For individualized guidance and modifications, speak with a dermatologist or nutritionist who specializes in managing eczema.

KNOWING INGREDIENTS AND LABELS ON FOOD

Search for foods labeled "hypoallergenic" or "eczema-friendly," but double-check by checking ingredients for potential irritants like artificial colors, preservatives, and common allergens like dairy, gluten, and nuts. When developing an eczema diet, it's important to navigate food labels and learn to identify common allergens and additives that may trigger skin reactions.

Learn about labels such as "organic," "natural," and "non-GMO," which can suggest better options but still need a careful reading of the ingredients list; become familiar with other names for allergens (milk, for example, can also be referred to as casein or whey) to prevent accidental exposure; and give preference to foods with fewer ingredients and less processing because these are less likely to cause flare-ups of eczema.

When in doubt, get in touch with the manufacturer to find out about ingredients or possible cross-contamination hazards. Make it a habit to regularly read labels because product formulations can change.

TIPS FOR GROCERY BUYING FOR ECZEMA-FRIENDLY FOODS

Effective grocery shopping for an eczema-friendly diet starts with careful planning and list-making. Examine your meal plan and decide which ingredients you'll need before you go. Focus on fresh produce, lean proteins, and whole grains; avoid processed foods that could contain allergens or additives. Shop at specialty stores or local farmers' markets; they often have organic and allergy-friendly products.

Keep an eye out for triggers like artificial flavors, colors, and preservatives by carefully reading product labels; choose products with few ingredients and those specifically labeled as safe for people with sensitive skin or eczema; and stock up on pantry staples like olive oil, nuts, and seeds that can be used as healthy substitutes in recipes.

Shop during off-peak hours to avoid crowds and give yourself more time for careful label reading. By implementing these tactics, you can prioritize foods that support your skin health and eczema management goals while streamlining your grocery shopping experience. Use bulk bins to buy grains, nuts, and seeds to save money and minimize packaging waste.

TECHNIQUES FOR MEAL PREPARATION IN A BUSY SCHEDULE

Maintaining an eczema-friendly diet requires meal preparation, which is especially important when managing a hectic schedule. Set aside time each week to plan and cook meals ahead of time, emphasizing wholesome, easy recipes that minimize triggers. You can save time by batch-cooking staples like grains, lean proteins, and roasted vegetables, which will make meal assembly easier throughout the week.

Invest in high-quality food storage containers (glass or BPA-free plastic) that keep food fresh and portable. Divide cooked meals into portion sizes for quick grab-and-go options; this will help you resist the urge to reach for less healthful options when time is short. Add variety to your meal prep by switching up the flavors and ingredients to avoid taste fatigue and guarantee balanced nutrition.

Try different cooking techniques, like baking, steaming, or slow cooking, to preserve nutrients without using too many fats or oils. Label containers with meal contents and expiration dates to stay organized and guarantee food safety. By following these meal prep tips, you can successfully manage a busy lifestyle while adhering to a consistent diet for eczema.

Sample meal plans and beginner-friendly recipes that focus on nutrition and skin health make it easy to start an eczema-friendly diet. Start your day with overnight oats for breakfast, topped with fresh berries and a drizzle of honey or maple syrup for natural sweetness. For lunch, tuck into a quinoa salad with mixed greens, avocado, cherry tomatoes, and grilled chicken or tofu dressed with lemon juice and olive oil.

Snack ideas: carrot sticks with hummus, apple slices with almond butter, or a handful of mixed nuts and seeds. Dinner ideas: bake salmon seasoned with herbs and served over steamed broccoli and quinoa. Water, herbal teas, or cucumber and mint-infused water can be used to stay hydrated throughout the day.

Try modifying these meal plans and recipes to your tastes and dietary requirements. Use seasonal produce and herbs to add flavor and provide necessary vitamins and minerals.

CHAPTER FOUR

ECZEMA-FRIENDLY SUBSTANCES

CRUCIAL ITEMS FOR A DIET FOR ECZEMA

A diet that is eczema-friendly emphasizes whole, unprocessed foods that are high in nutrients that support skin health and reduce inflammation. It also emphasizes the importance of fresh fruits and vegetables, especially those high in vitamins A, C, and E, which help repair skin tissue and protect against damage.

It also includes fatty fish, such as salmon and mackerel, which are rich in omega-3 fatty acids and have anti-inflammatory properties.

Nuts and seeds, particularly flaxseeds and chia seeds, are excellent sources of omega-3 fatty acids and zinc, which are vital for skin repair and maintenance. Including probiotics-rich foods like yogurt and kefir can improve gut health, which is often linked to skin conditions like eczema.

Whole grains, such as oats, quinoa, and brown rice, provide fiber and essential minerals that aid in reducing inflammation.

Focusing on a balanced diet that includes a variety of these nutrient-dense foods can help manage the symptoms of eczema and support overall skin health. Lean proteins, such as poultry, beans, and legumes, supply the necessary amino acids for skin repair and immune function. These proteins are essential for maintaining healthy skin and preventing flare-ups.

ITEMS TO STEER CLEAR OF WHEN MANAGING ECZEMA

Processed foods and foods high in sugar, like sweets, sodas, and baked goods, can worsen inflammation and eczema symptoms because they contain additives and preservatives that can cause allergic reactions or sensitivities in people with eczema. These foods should be avoided or limited as they can cause flare-ups of eczema.

For some eczema sufferers, dairy products—such as milk, cheese, and yogurt—can be problematic because they can trigger allergic reactions and inflammation, which can irritate the skin and cause flare-ups. It could be helpful to switch to plant-based dairy substitutes, such as almond milk or coconut yogurt, which are less likely to trigger negative reactions.

Identifying and avoiding these allergens through an elimination diet can help manage eczema. It is important to monitor how the body reacts to different foods and to consult with a healthcare professional or dietitian to create a personalized eczema-friendly diet plan that avoids these triggers. Common allergens like eggs, nuts, and shellfish can also trigger eczema symptoms in susceptible individuals.

USING FOODS THAT REDUCE INFLAMMATION

Including foods that reduce inflammation in the diet can help manage the symptoms of eczema significantly. For example, turmeric, a spice with strong anti-inflammatory qualities, can be added to soups, stews, and smoothies. Its active ingredient, curcumin, helps soothe irritated skin and reduce inflammation. Ginger, on the other hand, has antioxidant and anti-inflammatory qualities and can be used in teas, marinades, and stir-fries to help manage the symptoms of eczema.

Leafy greens like spinach, kale, and Swiss chard are also great options because they are full of vitamins, minerals, and antioxidants that help reduce inflammation and support healthy skin. Berries: Berries like blueberries, strawberries, and blackberries are rich in antioxidants and vitamins that help combat inflammation and support skin health. These can be consumed fresh, in smoothies, or as toppings for yogurt and cereal.

Incorporating green tea into daily meals can help manage eczema and improve overall skin health. Green tea is a potent anti-inflammatory food that can be included in the diet. It contains antioxidants and polyphenols that help reduce inflammation and protect the skin from damage.

Regularly drinking green tea or using it as a base for smoothies can provide these benefits.

HYDRATION'S PART IN TREATING ECZEMA

Drinking enough water throughout the day helps keep the skin hydrated and flushes out toxins that can exacerbate eczema symptoms. Aim for at least eight glasses of water per day, and increase intake during hot weather or after physical activity to compensate for lost fluids. Staying properly hydrated is essential for managing eczema and maintaining healthy skin.

Consuming high-water foods can help you stay hydrated even when you're not drinking a lot of water. Fruits and vegetables like celery, cucumbers, watermelon, and oranges are high in vitamins and minerals that support skin health and are great sources of hydration. You can include these foods in meals and snacks to help you stay hydrated.

Maintaining proper hydration through these methods is essential for managing eczema and promoting overall skin health. Using a humidifier in the home can also help keep the skin hydrated, especially in dry or cold climates. Humidifiers add moisture to the air, preventing the skin from drying out and reducing the risk of flare-ups. Applying moisturizers right after bathing while the skin is still damp can lock in moisture and provide a protective barrier against environmental irritants.

SUPPLEMENTAL DIETARY PRODUCTS FOR HEALTHY SKIN
Omega-3 fatty acid supplements, which are derived from fish oil or flaxseed oil and are known for their anti-inflammatory properties, can help reduce eczema symptoms. These supplements can be taken daily to ensure an adequate intake of omega-3s, especially for individuals who may not be getting enough through their diet. Nutritional supplements can play a supportive role in managing eczema and improving skin health.

Probiotics supplements can also be helpful, as they promote gut health, which is linked to skin conditions like eczema.

A healthy gut microbiome can improve immune function and reduce inflammation, thereby helping to manage eczema symptoms. Vitamin D is another essential nutrient for skin health, and a deficiency can worsen eczema symptoms. Wintertime is a good time to take vitamin D supplements to help maintain healthy skin.

A daily zinc supplement can help reduce flare-ups of eczema and promote healthy skin. It is important to speak with a healthcare provider before beginning any new supplement regimen to make sure it is right for you and to prevent any potential interactions with other medications or conditions. Zinc is essential for immune system function and wound healing.

CHAPTER FIVE

COOKING METHODS FOR A DIET AGAINST ECZEMA

OPTIMAL COOKING TECHNIQUES FOR PRESERVING NUTRIENTS

The key to cooking for eczema is to use methods that preserve as much of the nutrients as possible in your ingredients. One of the best ways to preserve vitamins and minerals in vegetables and proteins is to steam them. This helps to prevent the nutrient loss that can occur when boiling, as vitamins can leach into the water. Stir-frying is another great way to cook, as it uses high heat for a brief period, maintaining the nutritional integrity of vegetables while producing a tasty and quick meal. Roasting at lower temperatures can also caramelize the natural sugars in meats and vegetables without compromising their nutritional value.

Finally, consider sous-vide cooking, which involves vacuum-sealing food and cooking it in a water bath at precise temperatures. This method ensures that nutrients are locked in and flavors are enhanced without the need for added fats or high heat. For those who prefer a more hands-off approach, slow cooking can be very effective.

Using a slow cooker allows food to cook slowly over several hours, which helps retain nutrients that might be lost in high-heat cooking. This method is particularly good for making nutrient-rich broths and stews, which can form the basis for various eczema-friendly meals.

By incorporating these healthful cooking techniques into your meal preparation, you can help preserve vital nutrients while maintaining a delicious and eczema-friendly meal. By concentrating on these techniques, you can make a variety of meals that promote skin wellness and overall health, which will facilitate diet-based eczema management.

USING SPICES AND HERBS TO ADD FLAVOR WITHOUT GETTING RID OF THEM

Herbs and spices are a great way to flavor food without triggering the irritation that can aggravate eczema. You can use a lot of fresh herbs, such as basil, parsley, cilantro, and thyme, to make your food taste better. These herbs are not only flavorful, but they are also full of antioxidants and anti-inflammatory qualities. For example, you can add a lot of fresh basil to a salad or sprinkle chopped parsley over a dish right before serving.

Additionally, spices like turmeric, ginger, and cinnamon are excellent options. Turmeric has an ingredient called curcumin, which has potent anti-inflammatory properties that can help lessen flare-ups for eczema. Ginger is great for soups, stews, and teas; it also adds a warm, spicy note and aids in digestion. Cinnamon is another versatile spice that works well in both savory and sweet dishes, giving many eczema-friendly recipes a mild, sweet flavor.

When using dried herbs and spices, make sure they are pure and free of additives that could irritate the skin.

Mixing spices like cumin, coriander, and fennel seeds can result in a delicious blend that can be used in various dishes, from roasted vegetables to grilled meats. By focusing on natural, non-irritating herbs and spices, you can maintain a diverse and enjoyable diet without compromising the health of your skin. Making your spice blends can be a fun and effective way to ensure that your meals are flavorful and safe for an eczema diet.

ECZEMA-FRIENDLY RECIPES: SIMPLE AND QUICK

You can maintain your diet without spending too much time in the kitchen by making simple, quick, and easy eczema-friendly meals. One-pot meals are especially practical and can be loaded with healthy ingredients. For example, a quick, nutrient-dense meal can be made with quinoa and vegetable stir-fry dressed simply with olive oil, lemon juice, and fresh herbs.

Another simple, 30-minute meal is baked salmon with steamed broccoli and sweet potatoes.

Another easy and adaptable meal idea for people with eczema is a salad. Begin with a bed of leafy greens, such as spinach or arugula, and then top with a mix of colorful veggies, like bell peppers, cucumbers, and carrots. Add lean proteins, like grilled chicken or chickpeas, and drizzle with a vinaigrette made of olive oil, apple cider vinegar, and honey. These salads are not only easy to put together, but they're also a great source of vitamins and minerals that promote healthy skin.

Smoothies are a great option for a quick, eczema-friendly breakfast or snack. For a creamy, nutrient-dense smoothie, blend ingredients like spinach, avocado, banana, and a splash of almond milk. You can also add a handful of nuts or a scoop of protein powder for extra nutrition. These recipes are made to be quick, simple, and flexible so you can still enjoy tasty, healthful meals even on your busiest days.

TIPS FOR BATCH COOKING AND FREEZING

Making large batches of soups, stews, and casseroles and portioning them into individual containers before freezing can help you freeze food in bulk and ensure that you always have a healthy meal on hand. For example, making a large pot of chicken and vegetable soup and freezing it in individual servings can provide quick lunches or dinners throughout the week. Batch cooking can be a lifesaver for those managing an eczema diet, providing ready-to-eat meals that are nutritious and eczema-friendly.

Foods like cooked grains, roasted vegetables, and lean proteins can also be batch-cooked and stored in the freezer for easy meal assembly. Proper storage techniques are essential when freezing meals to preserve the quality and nutritional value of the food. Use airtight containers or heavy-duty freezer bags to prevent freezer burn and preserve freshness. Label each container with the date and contents, so you can easily keep track of what you have.

Gaining proficiency in batch cooking and freezing will streamline meal preparation and guarantee that you always have eczema-friendly options on hand. Thaw meals in the refrigerator overnight or use your microwave's defrost setting if you're in a hurry. Reheat gently on the stovetop or in the oven, avoiding high temperatures that can degrade nutrients.

COOKING FOR FAMILIES WITH VARIOUS NUTRITIONAL REQUIREMENTS

Cooking for a family with varying dietary requirements, such as an eczema-friendly diet, calls for careful preparation and adaptability. Begin by identifying staple ingredients and easily customizable meals, such as roasted chicken with vegetables, which can be customized by serving different sides or toppings. For example, one family member may like the chicken served with quinoa, a gluten-free grain, while another may prefer it served with mashed potatoes or a crisp salad. This allows everyone to share a meal while meeting individual dietary requirements.

Make meal components that are interchangeable so that everyone in the family can customize their plate to fit their dietary needs and preferences. For instance, prepare different proteins like grilled fish, tofu, and lean meats, along with a variety of vegetable dishes and grains. By using separate serving dishes for each component, you can also help prevent cross-contamination for those who have severe allergies or sensitivities.

HEALTHY BREAKFAST CHOICES FOR PEOPLE WITH ECZEMA

Eating a nutrient-dense breakfast can help control the symptoms of eczema. Oatmeal is an excellent option because it contains anti-inflammatory qualities that help calm the skin. To make a bowl of gluten-free oats, whisk together some water or dairy-free milk substitute (almond or oat milk works well). Garnish with antioxidant-rich fresh berries and a sprinkling of flaxseeds or chia seeds for an added dose of omega-3 fatty acids. Steer clear of sugary toppings and dairy products, as they can exacerbate flare-ups.

Another great option for breakfast is a vegetable omelet made with ingredients that are friendly to people with eczema. To make the omelet, add chopped spinach, bell peppers, and zucchini, which are rich in vitamins and minerals that support skin health. Cook the omelet in a small amount of olive oil or coconut oil to avoid unhealthy fats that can exacerbate inflammation.

Eggs are a good source of protein, but if you suspect an egg allergy, substitute with chickpea flour to make a "vegan omelet."

A simple and quick breakfast option is a smoothie bowl full of skin-loving nutrients. Simply blend a base of banana and spinach with a cup of unsweetened almond milk, then top with sliced kiwi, pumpkin seeds, and a handful of blueberries. These ingredients provide a combination of vitamins A, C, and E, all of which are essential for healthy skin. Including anti-inflammatory and nutrient-dense foods in your daily breakfast routine can help alleviate the symptoms of eczema.

HEALTHY SNACKS TO MINIMIZE SYMPTOMS OF ECZEMA

A handful of nuts, like walnuts or almonds, which offer healthy fats and protein, can be paired with fresh fruit, like apples and pears, to help keep blood sugar stable and prevent eczema flare-ups. This combination helps keep you fuller for longer and discourages the urge to snack on unhealthy options that could aggravate your eczema.

Another eczema-friendly snack is vegetable sticks with hummus. Made from chickpeas, hummus is rich in skin-supporting nutrients like folate and zinc. Choose or prepare hummus without added preservatives or excessive salt, as these can irritate the skin. Carrot, celery, and cucumber sticks are full of vitamins and fiber, and when dipped in store-bought or homemade hummus, they add a protein boost.

A savory option would be rice cakes with avocado on top. To get the most nutrients, choose whole grain or brown rice cakes. Spread a mashed avocado on top, then sprinkle with sea salt and a little turmeric for anti-inflammatory effects. This snack is not only delicious, but it also contains healthy fats and antioxidants that can help reduce the symptoms of eczema.

SMOOTHIE RECIPES LOADED WITH NUTRIENTS THAT LOVE YOUR SKIN

Smoothies are an easy way to incorporate multiple skin-beneficial ingredients into one meal or snack. For example, try making a green smoothie by blending spinach or kale with half an avocado, a banana, and a cup of coconut water. This combination provides a potent amount of potassium, healthy fats, and vitamins A, C, and E, all of which are known to support skin health and hydration.

A tablespoon of chia seeds can add omega-3 fatty acids and fiber, both of which are good for reducing inflammation and promoting overall skin health. Strawberries, blueberries, and raspberries can be combined with a handful of spinach and unsweetened almond milk for a berry boost. Berries are rich in antioxidants, which help shield the skin from damage.

A tropical smoothie made with mango, pineapple, and a tiny piece of fresh ginger is another good option for your skin.

The vitamin C content of mangoes and pineapples is important for the production of collagen and skin repair, and the anti-inflammatory properties of ginger can help reduce flare-ups of eczema. These fruits can be blended with coconut milk to create a creamy, refreshing drink that promotes skin health from the inside out.

Sweet potato chips are a great gluten-free and dairy-free snack option. Slice a sweet potato thinly, toss with a little olive oil and sea salt, and bake until crispy. Sweet potatoes are high in beta-carotene, which the body converts into vitamin A, promoting healthy skin. For those with eczema, gluten and dairy can occasionally trigger symptoms, so finding suitable snack alternatives is important.

Another fantastic snack that is free of gluten and dairy is chia seed pudding, which is made by combining three tablespoons of chia seeds with one cup of unsweetened almond milk, a teaspoon of honey or maple syrup, and refrigerating the mixture overnight to thicken. Rich in fiber and omega-3 fatty acids, chia seeds also support digestive health and reduce inflammation, two factors that are crucial for managing eczema.

Finally, roasted chickpeas make a crunchy, satisfying snack. Rinse and drain a can of chickpeas, toss with olive oil, sea salt, and your preferred spices, such as cumin or paprika, and roast in the oven until crispy. Chickpeas are high in protein and fiber without gluten or dairy, so they're a great way to maintain a healthy diet while also preventing eczema symptoms.

CONTROLLING CRAVINGS WITHOUT MAKING ECZEMA WORSE

Choose naturally sweet fruits like dates or figs, which are high in natural sugars and fiber and provide a satisfying sweetness without the inflammatory effects of refined sugar. Pair them with a few nuts to balance the sweetness with some healthy fats and protein. Controlling cravings can be difficult, especially when trying to manage eczema.

If you're in the mood for something salty, consider making your kale chips: tear the leaves into bite-sized pieces, toss with a little olive oil and sea salt, and bake until crispy.

Rich in vitamins A and C, which are essential for healthy skin, kale is a superfood; making chips at home helps you avoid the excess salt and preservatives that are frequently found in store-bought varieties.

If you're craving something creamy, grab a dairy-free yogurt made with almond or coconut milk and top it with fresh berries and a honey drizzle for extra sweetness and antioxidants. Probiotics are another benefit of dairy-free yogurts; a healthy gut can help reduce inflammation and improve skin conditions like eczema, so you can satisfy your cravings without aggravating your condition.

TASTY SALADS TO REDUCE ECZEMA

Finding tasty eczema salad recipes requires concentrating on ingredients that are both gentle and supportive of general health. Begin with a base of leafy greens, like spinach or kale, which are high in vitamins and antioxidants that support skin health. Next, add cucumber slices for moisture and anti-inflammatory qualities, followed by colorful bell peppers that supply vitamin C and aid in the fight against oxidative stress. Finally, add avocado for its healthy fats that hydrate the skin from the inside out.

Add lean proteins, like grilled chicken or tofu, to your salad for a flavor and nutrition boost. Add some seeds, like chia or flaxseed, to your salad for omega-3 fatty acids that support skin barrier function. Toss with a little olive oil and lemon juice for a zesty and hydrating finish. These combinations not only nourish your body but also help alleviate eczema symptoms by avoiding common triggers and promoting skin health through balanced nutrition.

When prepared properly, soups and stews can provide comfort and healing for skin prone to eczema. Start with a homemade vegetable broth base, simmered with anti-inflammatory spices like turmeric and ginger, which are known for their calming effects. Add veggies like sweet potatoes and carrots, which are high in beta-carotene and promote skin cell regeneration. Add lentils or beans for a plant-based protein that nourishes without aggravating eczema symptoms.

If you want to add protein, go for lean cuts of meat or seafood, but make sure to cook them slowly so they retain moisture and minimize potential triggers. Season lightly with sea salt and herbs like parsley or cilantro, but stay away from heavy creams or dairy-based broths that can aggravate eczema. These soups and stews are comforting and warming, but they also promote skin health because they are made with balanced, nourishing ingredients.

ONE-POT DINNERS FOR SIMPLE CLEANING

For people with eczema who would like to streamline their cooking, one-pot meals are a practical solution for hectic schedules and low cleanup. Look for recipes that combine grains, protein, and vegetables all in one pot, like quinoa with chicken and vegetables. To add flavor, sauté onions and garlic in olive oil first, then add diced chicken or tofu.

Add colorful veggies like bell peppers, zucchini, and cherry tomatoes for vitamins and antioxidants that support skin health. Season with herbs like thyme or rosemary for added flavor without relying on salt, which can dehydrate the skin. These one-pot meals not only simplify cooking but also ensure balanced nutrition that supports eczema management through wholesome ingredients cooked together to retain their natural benefits.

Add grains like quinoa or brown rice, which provide fiber and essential nutrients without triggering eczema flare-ups.

DINNER OPTIONS THAT ARE RICH IN PROTEIN AND PLANTS

For eczema management, opting for plant-based and high-protein dinner options can be helpful because they often contain nutrients that support skin health without causing flare-ups. High-protein and high-fiber legumes, like black beans or chickpeas, are gentle on sensitive skin and can be combined with quinoa or whole grains, like barley, for a complete amino acid profile that supports skin cell regeneration.

Add leafy greens, like spinach or kale, which are loaded with vitamins and minerals that support healthy skin function. Add some flavor with plant-based fats, like avocado or olive oil, which supply essential fatty acids that moisturize the skin from the inside out. These plant-based dinners not only fuel the body but also help control eczema symptoms by offering balanced nutrition free of common triggers.

SWEETS AND TREATS THAT WON'T CAUSE FLARE-UPS OF ECZEMA

For people with eczema, desserts, and treats can still be included in a balanced diet as long as they contain ingredients that promote skin health and reduce inflammation. Fruit-based desserts, like baked apples or poached pears, provide natural sweetness without the added sugars that exacerbate eczema. When baking, use oats or almond flour for a gluten-free option that is easier on the stomach and less likely to cause skin reactions.

If you're looking for a satisfying way to indulge while supporting skin health through thoughtful ingredient choices and mindful moderation, try using coconut or almond milk instead of cow's milk in recipes. You can also experiment with dark chocolate or carob chips for a decadent touch that provides antioxidants without dairy or excess sugar.

CHAPTER SIX

PARTICULAR DAYS AND HOLIDAYS

ORGANIZING ECZEMA-FRIENDLY EVENTS

When throwing an event for people who have eczema, you should make sure that everyone feels comfortable and included by talking to them about their dietary requirements and triggers. You should also plan a menu that includes fresh, whole foods like vegetables, lean proteins, and gluten-free grains, and steer clear of common allergens like dairy, nuts, and processed foods. You should also think about providing a variety of options, like a build-your-own salad or grain bowl station, where guests can customize their meals according to their preferences and restrictions.

Apart from the food itself, keep an eye out for potential allergens in the dining area, such as scented candles or flowers that might aggravate eczema symptoms. Provide hypoallergenic hand soaps and steer clear of strong-smelling cleaning products.

It's also important to create a stress-free atmosphere since stress can lead to flare-ups in eczema. Play soothing music, keep the temperature comfortable, and provide comfortable seating arrangements to help guests unwind and enjoy the occasion.

Fun non-food activities like board games, crafts, or outdoor activities like a nature walk can add to the enjoyment of the gathering and help to shift the focus away from food so that everyone can participate without feeling obligated to follow special dietary requirements. By considering your guests' needs and fostering a considerate, welcoming environment, you can successfully host an eczema-friendly gathering.

CUSTOMIZED HOLIDAY DISHES FOR ECZEMA DIETS

This means that you can make thoughtful adjustments and modifications to classic recipes to make traditional holiday meals safe for people with eczema. To start, identify common allergens in traditional dishes, such as dairy, gluten, and nuts, and find suitable alternatives.

For example, you can use seed-based spreads in place of nut butter, coconut or almond milk in place of dairy milk, and gluten-free flours in place of wheat flour.

A balanced, nutritious meal that supports overall skin health can be made by modifying cooking methods to make the meals as healthful as possible. For example, instead of frying, try baking, grilling, or steaming to cut down on the amount of added oils and fats that can exacerbate inflammation. When making holiday favorites like stuffing, pies, and casseroles, look for recipes that are specifically made to be allergen-free, or make your versions using ingredients that are friendly to eczema sufferers.

A holiday feast that everyone can enjoy without sacrificing taste or tradition can be created by following these simple steps: encourage guests to share their eczema-friendly recipes and experiences, fostering a sense of community and support; and use vibrant, seasonal produce to add color and appeal to your dishes, invitingly serving them.

It can be enjoyable and fulfilling to make eczema-friendly desserts for special occasions. To begin, look for recipes that call for natural sweeteners like honey, maple syrup, or coconut sugar rather than refined sugars, which can aggravate eczema symptoms and cause inflammation. For instance, a straightforward fruit salad topped with honey or a baked apple dessert can satiate sweet cravings without causing harm from processed sugars. Using gluten-free flours like almond, coconut, or oat flour can also help prevent flare-ups caused by gluten.

Use well-known ingredients to improve skin health: berries, which are high in antioxidants and can be used in smoothies, parfaits, or baked goods as toppings; coconut milk or yogurt, which can be used as excellent dairy-free bases for creamy desserts like puddings or ice creams; flaxseeds or chia seeds, which can be used as egg substitutes in baked goods to add a nutritional boost while binding the ingredients; these alternatives help produce moisturizing, delicious, and eczema-friendly cakes and cookies.

Dessert presentation is important. Make your eczema-friendly desserts stand out with vibrant fruits, edible flowers, and visually appealing plating. Highlight the flavors and health benefits of these healthier options to entice guests to try them. Experiment with different ingredients and preparation methods to create a range of delectable, eczema-safe desserts that will make any special occasion memorable and pleasurable.

ADVICE FOR EATING OUT WHILE TAKING CARE OF ECZEMA

When eating out, it's important to communicate clearly and plan. Look up safe options on the menu online before selecting a restaurant, and find out if they serve allergy-free meals. You can also call ahead and discuss your dietary requirements with the manager or chef, asking if they can fulfill any special requests, like having ingredient lists for their dishes or using separate cookware to prevent cross-contamination.

Being proactive about your needs will help to ensure a safer dining experience.

When ordering at a restaurant, be very explicit about the dietary restrictions you have. Choose dishes that are simple and have few ingredients, like grilled meats, steamed vegetables, or salads with olive oil and lemon juice, rather than complicated sauces or dressings that may contain hidden allergens. Don't be afraid to ask questions about the preparation process and request adjustments as necessary. Most restaurants will make accommodations for patrons with dietary needs as long as they are properly informed.

Bring necessary items (e.g., eczema creams or antihistamines) in case you have an allergic reaction; it's also a good idea to pack a small snack in case the restaurant doesn't fully meet your needs. By following these guidelines and exercising caution when making decisions, you can enjoy eating out without sacrificing your comfort or health.

For those who suffer from eczema, stress management is essential because stress can worsen symptoms. Begin by establishing reasonable expectations for the celebration and making self-care a priority. Set aside time for relaxing activities like meditation, deep breathing exercises, or a quick walk to help you decompress.

Create a pre-event routine that consists of moisturizing your skin, dressing comfortably, and getting ready for any medications or treatments that may be required.

Acknowledging your limits and avoiding overcommitting to activities or responsibilities can help you avoid increased stress and flare-ups. During the celebration, take breaks if you feel overwhelmed. Find a quiet place to relax and practice deep breathing or mindfulness techniques to regain composure. Light conversation or focusing on enjoyable activities can also help divert attention from stressful triggers.

You can enjoy celebrations while managing your eczema symptoms by implementing these strategies. After the celebration, take some time to decompress and practice self-care. Your body can recover from any stress experienced during the event with a soothing bath, a gentle skincare routine, or a restful night's sleep. Consider what went well and what could be improved for future gatherings to make stress management easier.

CHAPTER SEVEN

CHANGING YOUR LIFESTYLE TO MANAGE ECZEMA

THE VALUE OF STRESS REDUCTION IN THE TREATMENT OF ECZEMA

The body releases hormones like cortisol when under stress, which can exacerbate eczema symptoms and lead to inflammation. Therefore, incorporating stress-relieving practices like yoga, mindfulness meditation, and deep breathing exercises can help lower cortisol levels and reduce skin inflammation. These activities not only promote relaxation but also give one a sense of control over their health, which contributes to overall well-being.

Social support is crucial; talking to friends, family, or a therapist can help manage stress more effectively. Creating a balanced daily routine that includes time for relaxation and self-care is essential for managing stress and its impact on eczema. Hobbies and activities that bring joy and relaxation can also significantly impact stress levels. Simple activities like reading, painting, or spending time in nature can provide a mental break and reduce stress.

By prioritizing tasks and creating attainable goals, people can maintain a sense of accomplishment and control. Consistently practicing stress management techniques can build a resilient mindset, which can help to better manage eczema and improve quality of life. Overcommitting and feeling overwhelmed can exacerbate stress and eczema symptoms.

SKINCARE PRACTICES TO SUPPORT DIETARY ADJUSTMENTS

In addition to dietary modifications, a good skin care regimen is crucial for controlling eczema. Begin with a mild, fragrance-free cleanser to prevent skin irritation. After cleansing, use a thick, moisturizing cream or ointment to seal in moisture and shield the skin barrier. Ceramides, hyaluronic acid, and colloidal oatmeal are good for calming and hydrating skin that is prone to eczema.

Regular moisturizing is essential for keeping skin hydrated, especially after bathing. In dry environments, using a humidifier can also help keep skin hydrated. Hot showers should be avoided because they deplete the skin's natural oils, causing dryness and irritation. Instead, use lukewarm water and take short baths or showers. Pat dry with a soft towel and apply moisturizer right away to seal in moisture.

It's also important to protect the skin from potential irritants. To minimize irritation from clothing, wear soft, breathable materials like cotton. Choose hypoallergenic laundry detergents and fabric softeners instead of harsh ones.

Regular nail trimming and wearing gloves during activities that could irritate the skin can prevent scratching and further damage. Regular skincare routines along with dietary adjustments can greatly improve the health of the skin and reduce symptoms of eczema.

THE EFFECT OF EXERCISE ON ECZEMA SYMPTOMS

Physical activity increases blood circulation, which can help nourish the skin and promote healing; it also triggers the release of endorphins, the body's natural mood elevators, which can reduce stress and improve mental well-being; and finally, regular exercise can help manage weight, as obesity has been linked to increased eczema severity. Exercise is integral to managing eczema because it improves overall health and reduces stress.

Wearing loose, breathable clothing can help prevent irritation and excessive sweating, which can exacerbate eczema. When incorporating exercise, choose activities that minimize skin irritation. Low-impact exercises like walking, swimming, or yoga are excellent options. Swimming in chlorinated pools should be followed by a thorough rinse and application of moisturizer to prevent chlorine from drying out the skin.

Exercise can help manage eczema in many ways, improving both physical and mental health.

To prevent dehydration, it is important to stay hydrated during physical activity. Drink plenty of water before, during, and after. After working out, wash your skin gently with a fragrance-free cleanser to remove sweat and any possible irritants. Then, liberally apply moisturizer to your skin.

SLEEPING ENOUGH TO MAINTAIN SKIN HEALTH

A regular sleep schedule, which involves going to bed and waking up at the same time every day, can help improve sleep quality and support skin health. Sleep is essential for maintaining healthy skin because it allows the body to repair and regenerate.

Sleep deprivation can weaken immune system function, increase inflammation, and exacerbate eczema symptoms.

Establishing a pre-sleep routine, like taking a warm bath, practicing relaxation techniques, or reading, can signal the body that it's time to wind down. Limiting screen time before bed is also important, as blue light from screens can disrupt the sleep cycle. Comfortable, hypoallergenic bedding can reduce the risk of skin irritation. Overall, creating a sleep-friendly environment is essential.

Prioritizing sleep can lead to significant improvements in managing eczema and overall health. Managing nighttime itching can be difficult, but it's necessary for good sleep.

Keeping nails trimmed and wearing soft, breathable pajamas can help prevent scratching during sleep. If you need help, talk to your healthcare provider about medications or treatments for managing itching at night.

COMPREHENSIVE METHODS FOR HANDLING ECZEMA

Integrating natural remedies, such as herbal treatments and essential oils, can provide additional support. For example, chamomile and calendula have anti-inflammatory properties that can soothe irritated skin. Essential oils, such as lavender and tea tree oil, can be added to bath water or diluted in carrier oil for topical application to calm the skin and reduce inflammation. Holistic approaches to managing eczema consider the whole person, addressing physical, emotional, and environmental factors.

A key component of holistic eczema management is dietary modification. Anti-inflammatory foods like fruits, vegetables, nuts, and fatty fish can help lower systemic inflammation; avoiding trigger foods or known allergens like dairy, gluten, or processed foods can also help reduce symptoms; and probiotics and probiotics can help improve gut health, which is linked to skin health by promoting immune system function and maintaining a balanced microbiome.

Combining these holistic approaches with conventional treatments can provide a comprehensive strategy for managing eczema, and enhancing overall well-being and skin health.

Mind-body practices, like yoga, tai chi, and acupuncture, can help manage stress and promote relaxation.

These practices encourage mindfulness and balance, which can positively impact eczema symptoms. Regular mindfulness meditation practice can reduce stress, lower inflammation, and improve emotional resilience.

CHAPTER EIGHT

FAQS & TROUBLESHOOTING

HANDLING FLARE-UPS OF ECZEMA DESPITE DIETARY CHANGES

It's important to identify potential allergens or irritants that might be sneaking into your meals. Reading labels carefully and choosing fresh, whole foods can minimize the risk of hidden triggers. Keeping a detailed food diary to track what you eat and any subsequent reactions can help pinpoint specific foods that may be causing flare-ups. Eczema flare-ups can occur even when you follow an eczema-friendly diet, often due to individual variations.

Another crucial element is stress management since stress can worsen the symptoms of eczema. You can lower your stress levels and, as a result, the frequency and intensity of flare-ups by incorporating relaxation techniques like yoga, meditation, or regular exercise into your daily routine.

You can also maintain the health of your skin barrier by staying hydrated and applying moisturizer to your skin regularly.

Consultation with a healthcare professional may be necessary if flare-ups continue after dietary efforts have been made; they can conduct tests to identify particular food allergies or intolerances and offer advice on additional dietary modifications. In certain cases, additional treatments or medications may be needed to effectively manage severe symptoms.

TYPICAL OBSTACLES IN FOLLOWING AN ECZEMA DIET

Planning and preparing meals ahead of time and keeping eczema-friendly snacks on hand will help you resist the temptation of less healthy options. It also helps to inform friends and family about your dietary needs so they can support you in social situations. Adhering to an eczema diet can be difficult, especially with the temptation of comfort foods and social situations involving food.

Growing your herbs and vegetables can also be an inexpensive way to guarantee you have fresh, safe ingredients at your disposal. Purchasing in bulk, going to farmers' markets, and concentrating on seasonal produce are some ways to manage the potential increase in food costs that may arise from the need for specialty items or organic produce.

When it comes to restricted foods, cravings can be hard to control. One way to help you stay on track with your diet is to find appropriate replacements for the foods you crave. For example, if you're missing dairy, you can try almond or coconut milk. You can also experiment with different spices and herbs to add flavor to your food and make your diet more sustainable and enjoyable.

MODIFYING RECIPES TO SUIT INDIVIDUAL PREFERENCES IN TASTE

Long-term success requires modifying recipes to fit your taste preferences while following an eczema diet. Begin by figuring out what flavors and textures you love to eat, then look for eczema-friendly ingredients that can mimic those flavors and textures. For instance, if you enjoy creamy textures, avocado or coconut milk can be great alternatives to dairy products.

Trying out different cooking methods can also have a significant impact. For example, roasting vegetables can bring out their inherent sweetness, while grilling them can add a smoky flavor that enhances your meals. You can also add depth and complexity to your dishes without resorting to potentially irritating ingredients by using creative herb and spice combinations.

To help your palate adjust and find new favorite dishes that fit within your dietary guidelines, it's also helpful to gradually alter existing recipes rather than make drastic changes all at once.

HEALTHCARE EXPERT CONSULTATION FOR ECZEMA TREATMENT

When diet modifications are insufficient to effectively manage eczema, seeking advice from medical professionals is essential. Dermatologists, allergists, and dietitians can offer important insights into the condition and assist in creating a comprehensive management plan. They can perform tests to identify particular allergens or irritants and recommend appropriate treatments or dietary adjustments.

Having a multidisciplinary team approach can address various aspects of eczema, from skincare to nutrition and overall well-being. Frequent follow-ups with your healthcare team ensure that your management plan remains effective and can be adjusted as needed. They can also provide support and guidance on dealing with flare-ups, managing stress, and maintaining a balanced diet.

Apart from expert guidance, support groups, and forums can furnish useful advice and emotional support from peers going through comparable struggles. Reconnecting with a group of people who share your experience can be immensely comforting and give you extra incentive to adhere to your management plan.

It's common to feel overwhelmed by the limitations, but focusing on what you can eat instead of what you can't can make a significant difference. Emphasize the variety of safe and nutritious foods available, such as fresh fruits, vegetables, lean proteins, and whole grains. Addressing concerns about dietary restrictions is vital for maintaining a positive attitude towards an eczema-friendly diet.

Discovering delicious alternatives to restricted foods can also help ease concerns. For instance, quinoa, rice, and almond flour are just a few of the delectable gluten-free grains and flours available. Likewise, discovering new cuisines that naturally fit within your dietary restrictions can open your eyes to a whole new world of flavors and meal options.

A dietitian can provide personalized strategies to ensure you're meeting all your nutritional needs while adhering to your dietary guidelines.

CHAPTER NINE

PROLONGED ACHIEVEMENT AND UPKEEP

KEEPING AN EYE ON ECZEMA SYMPTOMS AND THE EFFECTS OF DIET

Understanding how different foods affect your skin condition and how they affect your eczema symptoms depends on keeping a detailed food diary, noting everything you eat and drink when you eat it, and any symptoms you experience. This will help you identify potential triggers and patterns, which will make it easier to steer clear of problematic foods in the future. It's important to pay attention to both immediate reactions and delayed symptoms, as some foods can affect your skin for hours or even days.

Apart from keeping a food journal, evaluate your skin condition regularly using a consistent technique, like taking pictures or assigning a number to each symptom's severity. This way, you can keep track of your progress and make educated diet choices.

Keep in mind that other variables can impact eczema, like stress, the environment, and skin care products; combining dietary data with these outside variables gives you a complete picture of what influences your eczema.

Frequent check-ins with a medical professional (dentist or nutritionist) can help you fine-tune your monitoring regimen even more. They can interpret your food diary and symptom logs, make dietary recommendations, and offer advice on how to manage eczema more successfully. These professionals can also recommend specific tests (allergy or food sensitivity tests) to identify triggers in your diet. By taking a proactive approach to monitoring, you can be sure you are making educated decisions and improving your eczema management over time.

REINTRODUCING FOODS FOLLOWING IMPROVEMENT IN SYMPTOMS

When you start to see improvements in your eczema symptoms, you can start the process of reintroducing foods to see which ones might be safe to eat. To start, pick one food that you have avoided and reintroduce it gradually, preferably with the help of a healthcare provider. Eat this food for three to five days while keeping an eye out for any flare-ups in your symptoms. Make thorough notes about your observations during this time in your food diary.

This methodical approach helps you accurately identify which foods are safe and which should be permanently avoided; if after the reintroduction period no symptoms appear, you can gradually increase the portion size and keep a close eye on things.

If symptoms do reappear, remove the food from your diet again and wait until your eczema has stabilized before trying a different food. Reintroducing foods one at a time helps ensure clear results and prevents confusion.

Patience is essential during this phase. Reintroducing foods too soon or in large quantities can result in flare-ups, making it challenging to identify safe options.

During this phase, always seek personalized advice and support from your healthcare provider. Their knowledge and experience can guide you through the reintroduction process more skillfully, ensuring that you sustain the progress you've made in controlling your eczema through diet.

CREATING A SUSTAINABLE LIFESTYLE THAT IS ECZEMA-FRIENDLY

A holistic approach to health and wellness is necessary to create a sustainable eczema-friendly lifestyle. Begin by including a range of nutrient-dense, anti-inflammatory foods in your diet, such as whole grains, fruits, vegetables, and healthy fats. These foods can help reduce inflammation and support overall skin health. Try different recipes and meal plans to keep your diet interesting and varied while making sure you get all the nutrients you need without feeling deprived.

A healthy lifestyle includes regular exercise, adequate hydration, and good sleep hygiene. Exercise can help reduce stress, which is known to exacerbate eczema while staying hydrated and getting enough sleep supports overall skin health. Incorporate stress-relieving activities like yoga, meditation, or mindfulness practices into your daily routine to further support your skin. These modifications can help you manage your eczema in addition to dietary changes.

Building this sustainable lifestyle takes time and effort, but the benefits of reduced eczema symptoms and improved overall health make it a worthwhile investment. Lastly, establish a skincare routine tailored to eczema-prone skin. Use gentle, fragrance-free products, moisturize regularly, and avoid known irritants. Consistent care and maintenance of your skin barrier can significantly reduce flare-ups and improve your quality of life.

HONORING SIGNIFICANT ACHIEVEMENTS IN ECZEMA CONTROL

Acknowledging and celebrating your progress is crucial to staying motivated and acknowledging the progress you've made with your eczema management. Try setting attainable goals, like going a week without flare-ups, attempting a new eczema-friendly recipe, or successfully reintroducing a food without symptoms. Reward yourself for these accomplishments with small treats, relaxing activities, or new skincare products.

Include loved ones in your festivities to create a network of people who understand and value your efforts. Tell them about your accomplishments and struggles, and allow them to share in your happiness. This kind of group support can help the journey feel less lonely and offer support during difficult times. Marking significant anniversaries with others also serves to raise awareness of eczema among those in your immediate vicinity, creating a more understanding and encouraging atmosphere.

Keeping track of your accomplishments and progress in a journal or on social media can also be very inspiring. It can be energizing to look back at where you were at the beginning and realize how far you've come. These records act as a reminder of your strength and accomplishments, inspiring you to stick to your eczema management plan and aim for even bigger goals.

RESOURCES FOR CONTINUING ASSISTANCE AND INSTRUCTION

Long-term success in managing eczema requires making use of resources for continuing education and support. Start by looking for reliable information sources, like books, medical websites, and eczema-specific support groups. These resources can offer current information on treatments, dietary recommendations, and coping mechanisms. Online forums and social media groups can also provide invaluable peer support by connecting you with people who can relate to your experiences and can offer guidance and encouragement.

Maintaining an open line of communication and scheduling regular check-ins with healthcare professionals is another crucial resource to help you stay on track with your eczema management. Dermatologists, allergists, and nutritionists can provide personalized guidance based on the latest research and your unique needs. They can help you develop and adjust your management plan as needed, ensuring you are always using the most effective strategies.

If you're interested in learning more about eczema and related topics, you should think about attending conferences, webinars, or educational workshops. These can help you gain a better understanding of the condition and expose you to new treatments and methods. By keeping up to date on eczema care advancements, you can also make informed decisions and modify your management plan as needed.

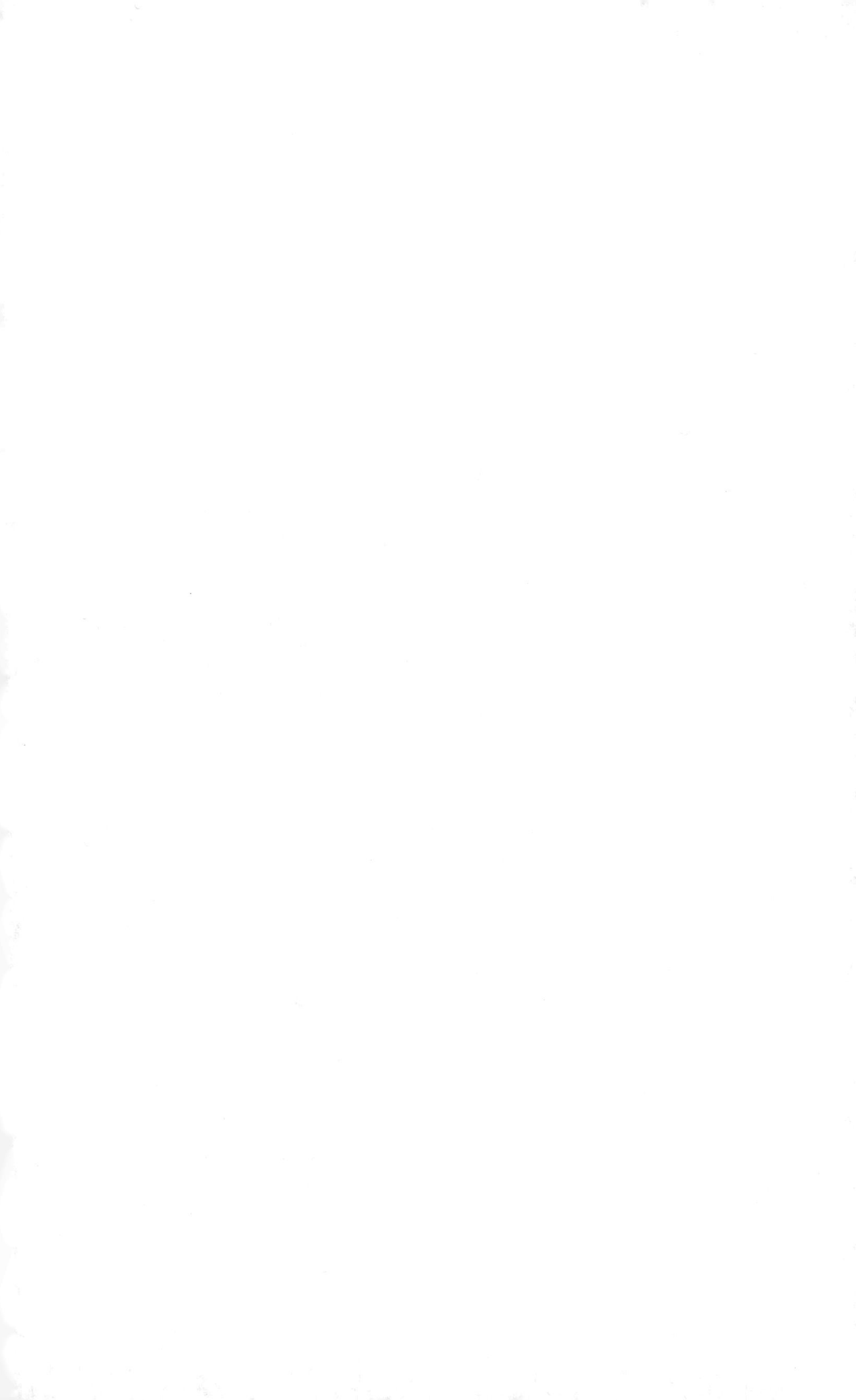

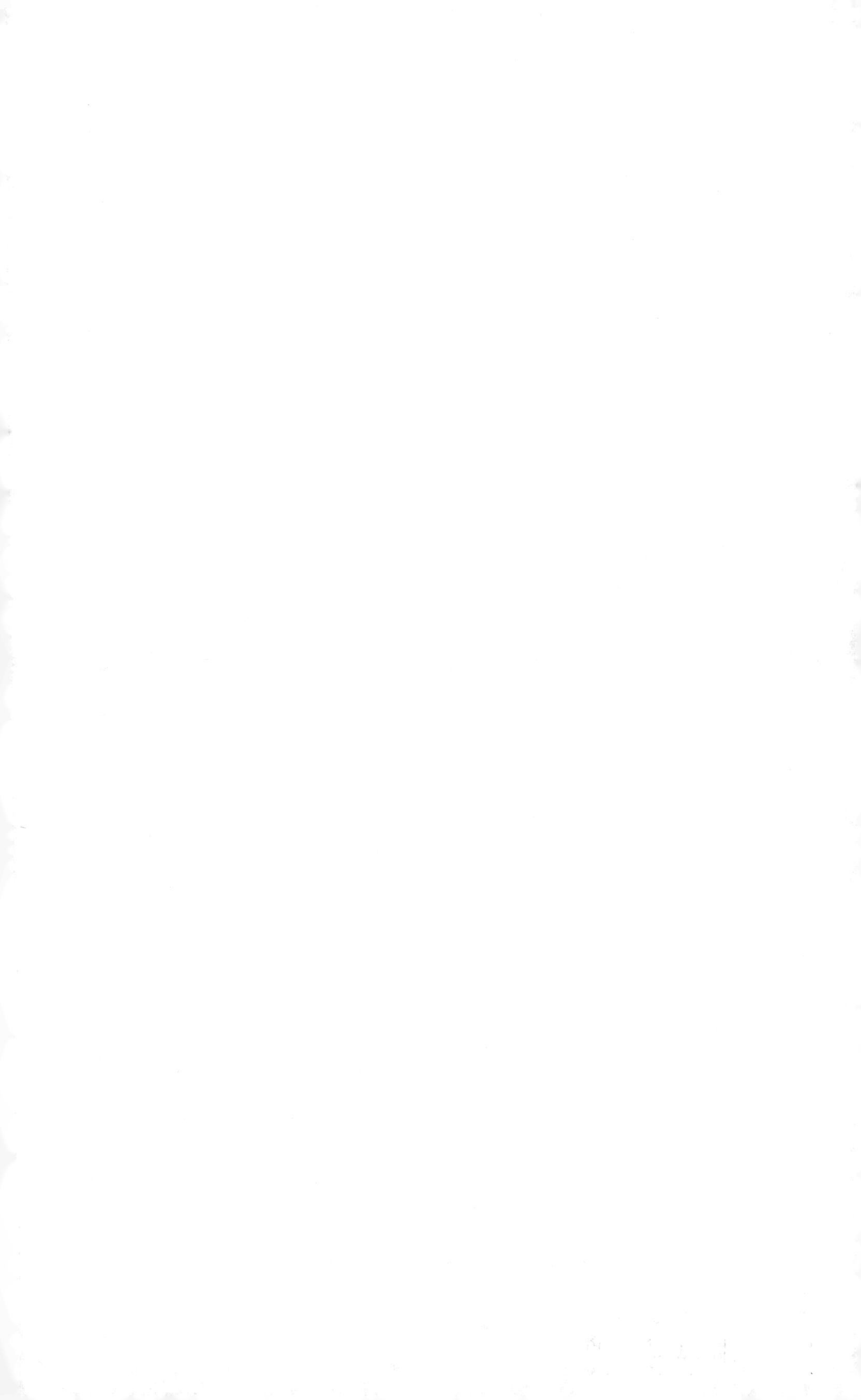